Instant Pot Cookbook 2021

Quick & Easy Recipes

Isabel Soto

© **Copyright 2021 - All rights reserved.**

The content contained within this book may not be reproduced, duplicated or transmitted without direct written permission from the author or the publisher.

Under no circumstances will any blame or legal responsibility be held against the publisher, or author, for any damages, reparation, or monetary loss due to the information contained within this book. Either directly or indirectly.

Legal Notice:

This book is copyright protected. This book is only for personal use. You cannot amend, distribute, sell, use, quote or paraphrase any part, or the content within this book, without the consent of the author or publisher.

Disclaimer Notice:

Please note the information contained within this document is for educational and entertainment purposes only. All effort has been executed to present accurate, up to date, and reliable, complete information. No warranties of any kind are declared or implied. Readers acknowledge that the author is not engaging in the rendering of legal, financial, medical or professional advice. The content within this book has been derived from various sources. Please consult a licensed professional before attempting any techniques outlined in this book.

By reading this document, the reader agrees that under no circumstances is the author responsible for any losses, direct or indirect, which are incurred as a result of the use of information contained within this document, including, but not limited to, — errors, omissions, or inaccuracies.

Sommario

Side Dishes 8

Tender Greens 8

Paprika Hash Brown 11

Wrapped Asparagus 14

Dill Rice...16

Orange & Carrot Puree 18

Beef Shumai 20

Black Beans Pasta 23

Creamy Cabbage Rice...25

Turnips Puree with Chives 27

Garlic Cauliflower Florets 29

Peppery Squash 31

Turmeric Mushrooms..33

Half and Half & Spinach 36

Garlicky Butternut Squash..38

Buttery Celery Cubes 40

Broccoli Garlic Mix 42

Coconut Zucchini Strips 44

Glazed Onion 47

Butter Spinach 50

Feta Beetroot Salad 52

Creamed Onions Halves 54

Cider Onions 57

Almond Tortillas 59

Zoodles 61

Romano Zucchini 63

Salty Spaghetti Squash 66

Mozzarella Zucchini Casserole 68

Button Beans Casserole 70

Ground Zucchini Casserole 72

Almons and Mozzarella Zucchini Strips 74

Cabbage Rice 77

Cheddar Creamy Gratin 79

White Onion Rings 81

Rosemary Halves 83

Sweet Baby Carrot 85

Chili Zucchini Bowl 87

Thyme Asparagus 90

Minced Radish 92

Peppery Cubes 94

Pecan Salad 96

Cheese Gnocchi 98

Purple Cabbage Steaks 101

Cauliflower and Goat Cheese 104

Mushrooms and Fall Vegetables 106

Garlic Broccoli 108

Tots with Broccoli 110

Vegetable Fritters 112

Pressured Asparagus 114

Roasted Cider Steak.. 116

Cayenne Pepper Green Beans 118

Introduction

This total as well as beneficial guide to immediate pot cooking with over 1000 dishes for breakfast, supper, supper, as well as also desserts! This is one of one of the most extensive split second pot recipe books ever before released thanks to its selection and exact instructions.

Ingenious dishes as well as classics, modern take on family's most liked meals-- all this is yummy, simple and obviously as healthy and balanced as it can be. Adjustment the method you prepare with these ingenious instant pot directions. Required a brand-new dinner or a treat? Here you are! Best immediate pot meals integrated in a couple of basic actions, even a beginner can do it! The instantaneous pot specifies the way you cook daily. This instant pot cookbook aids you make the outright most out of your weekly menu.

The only immediate pot book you will ever before require with the utmost collection of dishes will certainly help you towards a simpler as well as healthier kitchen area experience. If you wish to save time cooking dishes extra effectively, if you want to supply your family food that can please also the pickiest eater, you remain in the best place! Master your instant pot as well as make your cooking needs suit your active way of living.

Side Dishes

Tender Greens

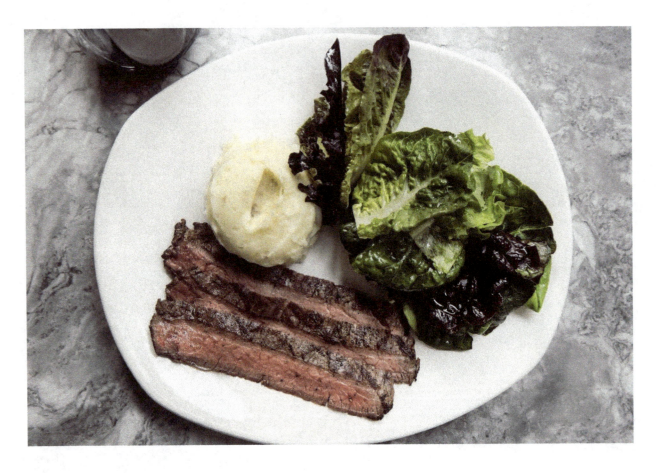

Prep time: 10 minutes

Cooking time: 20 minutes

Servings: 2

Ingredients:

- 2 cups collard greens, chopped
- ½ cup of water
- 3 tablespoons heavy cream
- 1 teaspoon salt
- 1 teaspoon paprika
- ¼ cup walnuts, chopped

Directions:

1. Place collard greens in the cooker.
2. Sprinkle the greens with salt and paprika. Add heavy cream and water.
3. Mix up the greens gently and close the lid. Cook them for 3 minutes on High-pressure mode.
4. Then allow natural pressure release for 10 minutes.

5. Open the lid and add walnuts. Mix up the meal and transfer on the serving plates.

Nutrition: calories 190, fat 18, fiber 3, carbs 5.3, protein 5.4

Paprika Hash Brown

Prep time: 15 minutes

Cooking time: 13 minutes

Servings: 6

Ingredients:

- 1-pound white cabbage, shredded
- 1 white onion, diced
- 1 tablespoon apple cider vinegar
- 1 teaspoon salt
- 1 teaspoon ground black pepper
- 3 oz bacon, chopped
- 1 cup heavy cream
- ½ cup of water

- ½ teaspoon tomato paste
- 1 teaspoon paprika
- 1 garlic clove, diced
- 1 oz pork rinds

Directions:

1. Put the shredded cabbage in the mixing bowl. Sprinkle it with apple cider vinegar, salt, ground black pepper, and paprika.

2. Mix up well and leave the mixture for 10 minutes.

3. After this, transfer it in the cooker.

4. Add chopped bacon, heavy cream, water, tomato paste, garlic clove, and pork rinds. Mix it up carefully and close the lid.

5. Cook the hash brown on High-pressure mode for 13 minutes. Then allow natural pressure release for 10 minutes. Open the lid and mix up the meal well.

Nutrition: calories 202, fat 15.2, fiber 2.5, carbs 7.6, protein 10

Wrapped Asparagus

Prep time: 10 minutes

Cooking time: 7 minutes

Servings: 4

Ingredients:

- 1-pound asparagus
- 7 oz bacon, sliced
- ½ teaspoon salt
- 1 teaspoon olive oil
- ½ teaspoon cayenne pepper

Directions:

1. Sprinkle the sliced bacon with salt, cayenne pepper, and olive oil.

2. Then wrap asparagus into the sliced bacon and place in the cooker basket.

3. Lower the air fryer lid and cook the side dish for 7 minutes. The cooked meal should have crispy bacon.

Nutrition: calories 302, fat 22.1, fiber 2.4, carbs 5.2, protein 20.9

Dill Rice

Prep time: 10 minutes

Cooking time: 5 minutes

Servings: 4

Ingredients:

- 1 ½ cup cauliflower
- 1 cup of water
- 1 tablespoon butter
- ¼ cup heavy cream
- 1 tablespoon dried dill
- 1 teaspoon salt

Directions:

1. Chop the cauliflower roughly and transfer it into the food processor.

2. Blend the vegetables until you gets cauliflower rice. Place the "cauliflower rice" in the cooker.

3. Add butter, salt, dried dill, heavy cream, and water.

4. Close and seal the lid. Cook the meal on High-pressure mode for 5 minutes. Use quick pressure release.

5. Open the lid and stir the cauliflower rice carefully.

Nutrition: calories 63, fat 5.7, fiber 1.1, carbs 2.6, protein 1.1

Orange & Carrot Puree

Prep time: 15 minutes

Cooking time: 25 minutes

Servings: 6

Ingredients:

- 5 medium carrots
- ½ cup of water
- ½ cup of orange juice
- 1 teaspoon butter
- ½ teaspoon cinnamon

Directions:

1. Wash the carrots and peel them.

2. Slice the carrots and place them in a mixing bowl. Sprinkle the vegetables with cinnamon and mix well.

3. Leave the mixture for 10 minutes to get the carrot juice.

4. Transfer the mixture with the liquid in the pressure cooker. Add water and orange juice. Close the lid, and set the pressure cooker mode to "Sauté."

5. Cook for 25 minutes or until the carrots are soft.

6. Let the carrots rest briefly and transfer the mixture to a blender.

7. Blend well until smooth. Add butter and stir. Serve the carrot puree warm.

Nutrition: calories 36, fat 0.7, fiber 1.4, carbs 7.3, protein 0.6

Beef Shumai

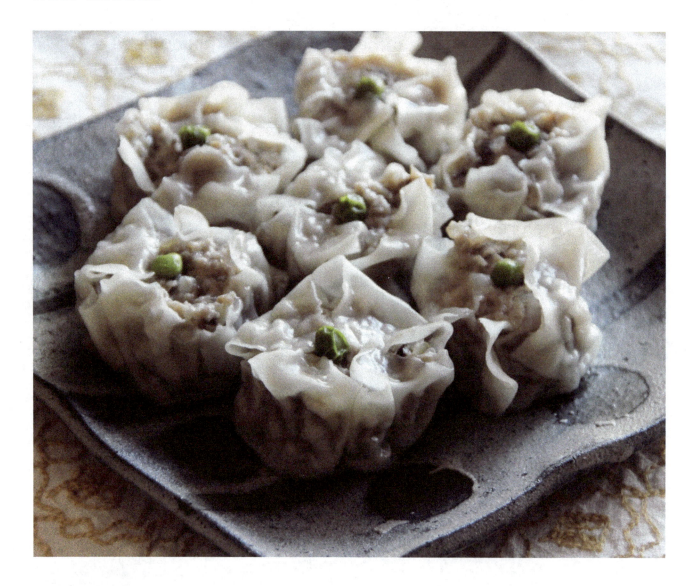

Prep time: 20 minutes

Cooking time: 10 minutes

Servings: 7

Ingredients:

- 6 ounces wonton wraps
- 1 cup ground beef
- 6 ounces tiger shrimp
- 1 teaspoon salt
- 2 tablespoons fish sauce
- ⅓ cup of soy sauce
- 1 teaspoon ground ginger
- 1 teaspoon white pepper
- 1 teaspoon salt
- ½ teaspoon cilantro
- 3 ounces green onions
- 1 teaspoon oregano
- 2 teaspoons ground white pepper

Directions:

1. Combine the ground beef, salt, cilantro, and oregano together.

2. Mince the tiger shrimp. Combine the minced shrimp with the ground white pepper.

3. Chop the green onion and add it to the shrimp mixture. Add the fish sauce, soy sauce, and ground ginger.

4. Combine the shrimp mixture and the ground beef mixture together. Mix well until combined completely.

5. Place the meat mixture into the wonton wraps and wrap the shumai to get the open top. Pour water in the pressure cooker.

6. Place the shumai in the steamer and transfer it to the pressure cooker.

7. Close the pressure cooker lid and cook the shumai for 5 minutes at the "Steam" mode.

8. After 10 minutes, release the steam and remove the dish from the pressure cooker and serve.

Nutrition: calories 142, fat 3, fiber 1, carbs 19.68, protein 9

Black Beans Pasta

Prep time: 10 minutes

Cooking time: 8 minutes

Servings: 6

Ingredients:

- 7 oz black beans pasta
- 1 cup of water
- 1 tablespoon rice vinegar
- 1 teaspoon Erythritol
- 1 teaspoon sesame seeds
- 1 teaspoon red chili flakes
- 1 teaspoon salt

Directions:

1. Place black beans pasta in the cooker.

2. Add water, salt, and chili flakes. Close and seal the lid.

3. Cook the pasta for 8 minutes in High-pressure mode. Then use quick pressure release and open the lid.

4. Drain water and transfer pasta in the bowl. In the separated bowl, mix up together rice vinegar, Erythritol, and sesame seeds. Stir gently.

5. Add the mixture into the pasta and shake gently. Transfer the meal into the serving bowls.

Nutrition: calories 111, fat 1.4, fiber 7.2, carbs 10.2, protein 14.9

Creamy Cabbage Rice

Prep time: 15 minutes

Cooking time: 3 minutes

Servings: 2

Ingredients:

- 8 oz white cabbage
- ½ cup of water
- ¾ cup cream
- 1 teaspoon salt

Directions:

1. Shred the cabbage until you get the cabbage rice mixture.

2. Add salt and mix up it well. Then transfer the cabbage rice in the Pressure cooker. Add water and cream. Mix it up. Close and seal the lid.

3. Cook the cabbage rice for 3 minutes on High-pressure mode.

4. Then allow natural pressure release for 10 minutes.

5. Open the lid and transfer hot cabbage rice into the serving bowls.

Nutrition: calories 86, fat 5.1, fiber 2.8, carbs 9.4, protein 2.2

Turnips Puree with Chives

Prep time: 10 minutes

Cooking time: 6 minutes

Servings: 4

Ingredients:

- 2 cups turnips, peeled, chopped
- 2 tablespoons chives, chopped
- 1 tablespoon butter
- 3 cups of water
- 1 teaspoon salt
- 1 teaspoon garlic powder

Directions:

1. Put turnip in the cooker. Add water and salt. Cook it on High-pressure mode for 6 minutes. Then use quick pressure release.

2. Open the lid and drain water. Transfer turnip into the food processor.

3. Add butter and garlic powder.

4. Blend it until you get smooth mash.

5. Transfer the turnip mash in the serving bowls and sprinkle with chives. Mix up the meal gently.

Nutrition: calories 63, fat 2.9, fiber 2.1, carbs 8.6, protein 1.2

Garlic Cauliflower Florets

Prep time: 15 minutes

Cooking time: 5 minutes

Servings: 6

Ingredients:

- 15 oz cauliflower florets
- 1 teaspoon salt
- 1 tablespoon garlic powder
- 1 tablespoon avocado oil
- 1 teaspoon butter, melted
- ½ teaspoon dried oregano

Directions:

1. Mix up together salt, garlic powder, avocado oil, melted butter, and dried oregano.

2. Brush every cauliflower floret with the garlic mixture and leave for 10 minutes to marinate. After this, transfer the vegetables in the cooker basket.

3. Sprinkle them with the remaining garlic mixture.

4. Lower the crisp lid and cook the cauliflower for 5 minutes or until it starts to get light brown color and tender texture.

5. Transfer the side dish on the serving plates.

Nutrition: calories 31, fat 1, fiber 2.1, carbs 5, protein 1.7

Peppery Squash

Prep time: 15 minutes

Cooking time: 10 minutes

Servings: 3

Ingredients:

- 10 oz spaghetti squash
- 1 tablespoon butter
- 1 teaspoon ground black pepper
- 1 cup water, for cooking

Directions:

1. Pour water in the cooker and insert trivet inside.

2. Cut the spaghetti squash into halves and remove seeds. Place the squash on the trivet. Close and seal the lid.

3. Cook the vegetable on High-pressure mode 10 minutes. Then make a quick pressure release. Open the lid.

4. Transfer the spaghetti squash on the plate and shred the flesh with the help of the fork. You will get the spaghetti shape mixture.

5. Sprinkle it with ground black pepper and add butter. Stir it well. It is recommended to serve the side dish warm or hot.

Nutrition: calories 65, fat 4.4, fiber 0.2, carbs 7, protein 0.7

Turmeric Mushrooms

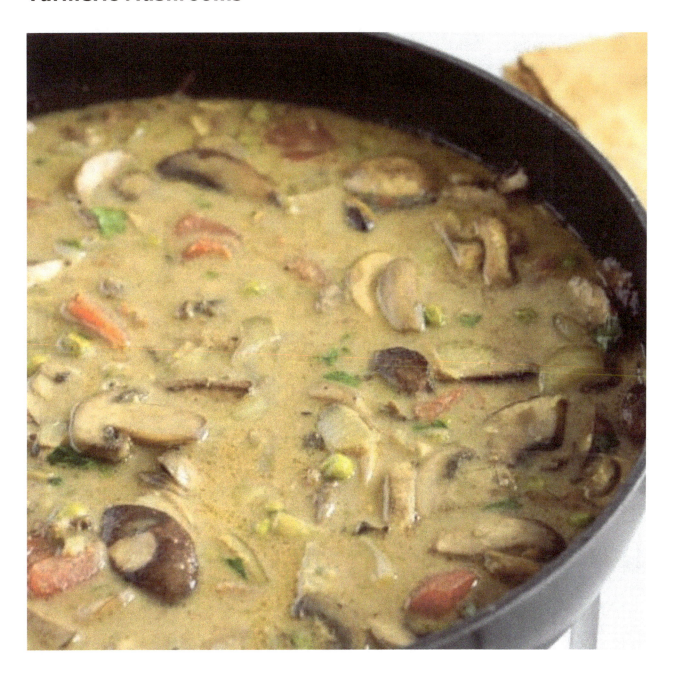

Prep time: 15 minutes

Cooking time: 25 minutes

Servings: 6

Ingredients:

- 2 tablespoons turmeric
- 1 tablespoon garlic powder
- 1 teaspoon minced garlic
- 1 teaspoon of sea salt
- ½ cup parsley
- 1 tablespoon olive oil
- 1 tablespoon butter
- 10 ounces large mushroom caps

Directions:

1. Wash the mushroom caps and remove the stems and gills.

2. Wash the parsley and chop it with the mushroom stems. Place the parsley in a blender and pulse several times.

3. Transfer the blended parsley in the mixing bowl. Add butter, minced garlic, sea salt, garlic powder, and turmeric. Stir the mixture well until smooth.

4. Fill the mushroom caps with the parsley mixture. Spray the pressure cooker with the olive oil inside and transfer the mushroom hat there.

5. Close the lid and cook on the "Sear/Sauté" mode for 25 minutes.

6. When the cooking time ends, open the lid and leave the mushroom caps in the machine for 5 minutes.

7. Remove the mushroom caps from the pressure cooker and serve.

Nutrition: calories 66, fat 4.5, fiber 0.8, carbs 4.3, protein 2

Half and Half & Spinach

Prep time: 10 minutes

Cooking time: 13 minutes

Servings: 5

Ingredients:

- 3 cups spinach
- 1 cup half and half
- 1 teaspoon olive oil
- 1 teaspoon cilantro
- ½ teaspoon rosemary
- 1 tablespoon butter
- 1 teaspoon kosher salt
- 1 lemon

Directions:

1. Wash the spinach and chop it. Pour olive oil into the pressure cooker and preheat it on the "Sauté" mode.

2. Transfer the chopped spinach in the pressure cooker. Sprinkle it with kosher salt, rosemary, and cilantro.

3. Stir the mixture and sauté it for 3 minutes. Stir the mixture frequently.

4. Add the butter and half and a half.

5. Close the lid and cook the spinach on the "Sauté" mode for 10 minutes. Squeeze the lemon juice onto the spinach and mix well.

6. Remove the dish from the pressure cooker and rest briefly. Transfer it to serving plates.

Nutrition: calories 99, fat 8.9, fiber 0.8, carbs 3.9, protein 2.1

Garlicky Butternut Squash

Prep time: 10 minutes

Cooking time: 15 minutes

Servings: 4

Ingredients:

- 1 pound butternut squash
- 1 tablespoon minced garlic
- 3 tablespoons butter
- ½ teaspoon white pepper
- 1 teaspoon paprika
- 1 teaspoon olive oil
- 1 teaspoon turmeric

Directions:

1. Wash the squash and make the thin incisions.

2. Melt the butter and combine it with the minced garlic and stir the mixture. Spray the pressure cooker with the olive oil inside.

3. Place the squash in the pressure cooker.

4. Sprinkle the squash with turmeric and paprika. Top it with garlic butter. Close the lid and cook the dish on the "Pressure" mode for 15 minutes.

5. When the cooking time ends, the butternut squash should be soft. Remove it from the pressure cooker and let it cool briefly before serving.

Nutrition: calories 145, fat 10, fiber 3, carbs 14.99, protein 2

Buttery Celery Cubes

Prep time: 10 minutes

Cooking time: 8 minutes

Servings: 6

Ingredients:

- 12 oz celery root, peeled
- 1 teaspoon salt
- 1 teaspoon ground black pepper
- 1 tablespoon butter
- 1 teaspoon olive oil
- 1 teaspoon minced garlic
- 1 tablespoon fresh parsley, chopped
- ¾ cup heavy cream

Directions:

1. Chop the celery root into medium cubes.

2. Preheat Foodi Cooker on Saute mode well. Then add butter and olive oil.

3. Preheat the mixture.

4. Add chopped celery root, ground black pepper, salt, and minced garlic.

5. Stir well and saute for 5 minutes. After this, add chopped parsley and heavy cream. Stir the mixture well.

6. Close the lid and cook it on High-pressure mode for 3 minutes.

7. Then allow natural pressure release for 10 minutes.

8. Chill the cooked celery cubes till the room temperature.

Nutrition: calories 101, fat 8.4, fiber 1.1, carbs 6.1, protein 1.3

Broccoli Garlic Mix

Prep time: 10 minutes

Cooking time: 10 minutes

Servings: 6

Ingredients:

- 1 white onion
- 1 pound broccoli
- ½ cup chicken stock
- 1 tablespoon salt
- 1 teaspoon olive oil
- 1 teaspoon garlic powder
- 3 tablespoons raisins
- 2 tablespoons walnuts, crushed

- 1 teaspoon oregano

- 1 tablespoon lemon juice

Directions:

1. Wash the broccoli and separate into small florets. Place the broccoli in the pressure cooker and sprinkle with the salt.

2. Close the lid and cook the vegetables on the "Pressure" mode for 10 minutes. Transfer the broccoli to a serving bowl.

3. Peel the onion and slice it. Add the onion to the broccoli.

4. Sprinkle the mixture with the garlic powder, oregano, crushed walnuts, raisins, and lemon juice.

5. Add olive oil and stir gently before serving.

Nutrition: calories 68, fat 3, fiber 3, carbs 4.09, protein 4

Coconut Zucchini Strips

Prep time: 10 minutes

Cooking time: 5 minutes

Servings: 6

Ingredients:

- 2 tablespoons sesame oil
- 3 green zucchini
- 1 tablespoon cilantro
- 1 teaspoon basil
- 1 tablespoon kosher salt
- 1 tablespoon butter
- ½ cup pork rinds
- ½ cup of coconut milk

- 4 eggs

- 1 tablespoon cumin

Directions:

1. Wash the zucchini and cut them into the strips.

2. Place the zucchini strips in the mixing bowl. Sprinkle them with the kosher salt, basil, and cilantro and stir the mixture.

3. Pour the sesame oil in the pressure cooker and preheat it on the "Sauté" mode.

4. Combine the eggs and coconut milk and whisk the mixture. Dip the zucchini strips in the egg mixture.

5. Coat the vegetables in the pork rind.

6. Place the zucchini strips in the pressure cooker and sauté them for 1 minute on each side. Sprinkle the dish with cumin and serve.

Nutrition: calories 225, fat 18.5, fiber 1.6, carbs 3.8, protein 12.4

Glazed Onion

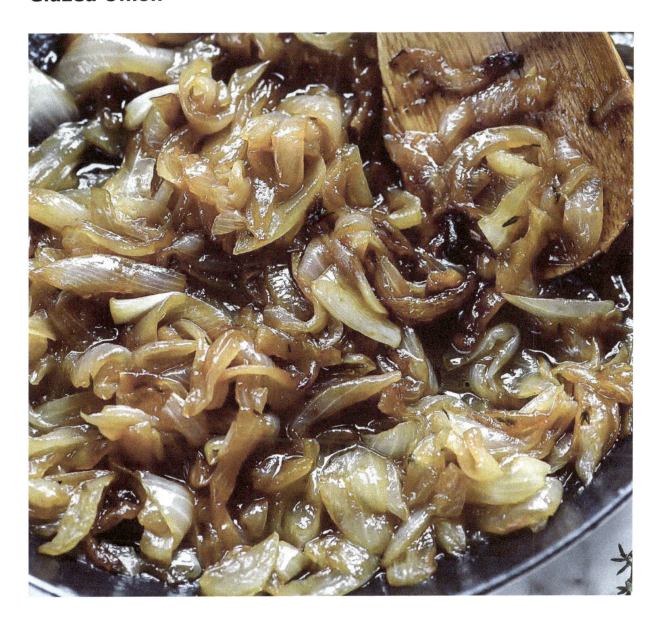

Prep time: 5 minutes

Cooking time: 12 minutes

Servings: 6

Ingredients:

- 1 pound white onions
- 3 tablespoons butter
- ⅓ cup Erythritol
- 1 teaspoon thyme
- ½ teaspoon white pepper
- 1 tablespoon paprika
- ¼ cup cream

Directions:

1. Peel the onions and slice them. Sprinkle the sliced onions with Erythritol.

2. Add thyme, white pepper, and paprika and stir the mixture. Place the onion mixture in the pressure cooker.

3. Add butter and set the pressure cooker to "Sauté" mode and sauté the mixture for 7 minutes.

4. Stir it frequently using a wooden spoon. Add cream and blend well.

5. Close the lid and cook the glazed onion at the pressure mode for 5 minutes.

6. Remove the cooked onions from the pressure cooker, allow it to rest briefly before serving.

Nutrition: calories 92, fat 6.6, fiber 2.2, carbs 8.2, protein 1.2

Butter Spinach

Prep time: 10 minutes

Cooking time: 10 minutes

Servings: 4

Ingredients:

- 4 cups spinach, chopped
- 1 tablespoon butter
- 1 cup cream
- 1 teaspoon salt
- 4 oz Cheddar cheese, shredded
- 1 teaspoon cayenne pepper
- 1 teaspoon paprika
- 1 tablespoon olive oil

Directions:

1. Pour cream in the cooker. Add salt, butter, cayenne pepper, and paprika.

2. Preheat it on saute mode. When the liquid starts to boil, add chopped spinach.

3. Stir well and saute the greens for 5 minutes.

4. After this, sprinkle the spinach with shredded cheese and stir well. Close the lid and saute the meal for 5 minutes more.

5. Switch off Foodi Pressure cooker and open the lid. Mix up the spinach well.

Nutrition: calories 218, fat 19.4, fiber 1, carbs 3.9, protein 8.6

Feta Beetroot Salad

Prep time: 10 minutes

Cooking time: 35 minutes

Servings: 7

Ingredients:

- 1 pound beetroot
- 1 red onion
- 3 tablespoons sunflower oil
- 1 tablespoon pumpkin seeds
- 8 ounces feta cheese
- 1 tablespoon basil
- ½ cup fresh parsley
- 4 cups of water

Directions:

1. Peel the beetroot and place it in the pressure cooker.

2. Add water and close the lid. Cook the beetroot on manual mode for 35 minutes. Meanwhile, peel the onion and slice it.

3. Crumble the cheese and chop the parsley. When the beetroot is cooked, remove it from the pressure cooker and chill well.

4. Chop it into the medium cubes. Combine the beetroot with the sliced onion. Add pumpkin seeds and crumbled feta cheese. Sprinkle the mixture with basil and sunflower oil. Stir the salad well and transfer it to serving plate.

Nutrition: calories 180, fat 13.6, fiber 2, carbs 9.42, protein 6

Creamed Onions Halves

Prep time: 10 minutes

Cooking time: 25 minutes

Servings: 10

Ingredients:

- 1 cup cream
- 1 cup of coconut milk
- 6 big white onions
- 1 teaspoon ground black pepper
- ½ tablespoon salt
- 1 tablespoon paprika
- ½ cup fresh dill
- ½ cup basil

- 1 tablespoon cilantro

- 1 teaspoon mint

- 1 teaspoon minced garlic

Directions:

1. Peel the onions and slice them into thick slices.

2. Place the sliced onion in the pressure cooker. Combine the coconut milk and cream together in a mixing bowl.

3. Add ground black pepper, salt, and paprika and stir the mixture.

4. Add the cilantro, mint, and minced garlic. Stir the mixture well. Pour the cream mixture onto the onion slices.

5. Wash the fresh dill and basil and chop them. Sprinkle the onions with the chopped seasonings.

6. Close the pressure cooker lid, and set the pressure cooker mode to "Sauté". Cook the onions for 25 minutes or until soft.

7. Release the pressure and open the pressure cooker lid. Transfer the onions in the serving plates and sprinkle them with the gravy.

Nutrition: calories 116, fat 7.4, fiber 3.2, carbs 12.5, protein 2.4

Cider Onions

Prep time: 10 minutes

Cooking time: 17 minutes

Servings: 4

Ingredients:

- 4 medium white onion
- 1 tablespoon ground black pepper
- 2 tablespoons lemon juice
- 1 tablespoon apple cider vinegar
- 1 teaspoon Erythritol
- ½ teaspoon salt
- ½ teaspoon oregano
- 1 tablespoon olive oil

Directions:

1. Peel the onions and chop the vegetables roughly.

2. Combine the ground black pepper, Erythritol, salt, and oregano together in a mixing bowl and stir the mixture.

3. Sprinkle the chopped onions with the spice mixture and stir using your hands. Add the onions to the pressure cooker.

4. Sprinkle the mixture with the olive oil and set the pressure cooker to "Sauté" mode. Sauté the onions for 10 minutes. Stir them frequently.

5. Add apple cider vinegar and lemon juice, stir the mixture and sauté the dish for 7 minutes with the lid closed.

6. Remove the dish from the pressure cooker, let it rest briefly, and serve.

Nutrition: calories 81, fat 3.7, fiber 2.9, carbs 11.6, protein 1.5

Almond Tortillas

Prep time: 10 minutes

Cooking time: 6 minutes

Servings: 4

Ingredients:

- 1 cup almond flour
- ½ cup coconut flour
- ½ teaspoon salt
- 3 tablespoons olive oil
- ½ cup of water

Directions:

1. In the mixing bowl, mix up together almond flour, coconut flour, salt, and water. Stir the mixture with the help of spoon/fork until it is homogenous.

2. Then add olive oil and knead a non-sticky soft dough. Cut it into 4 pieces. Roll up every dough piece with the help of the rolling pin.

3. In the end, you should get 4 rounds (tortillas).

4. Preheat cooker on saute mode well. Place 1 tortilla in the cooker and cook it for 1 minute from each side.

5. Repeat the same steps with the remaining tortillas.

6. Cover the cooked tortillas with the towel to save them fresh.

Nutrition: calories 330, fat 27.5, fiber 8, carbs 13, protein 2

Zoodles

Prep time: 10 minutes

Cooking time: 10 minutes

Servings: 6

Ingredients:

- 2 medium green zucchini
- 1 tablespoon wine vinegar
- 1 teaspoon white pepper
- ½ teaspoon cilantro
- ¼ teaspoon nutmeg
- 1 cup chicken stock
- 1 garlic clove

Directions:

1. Wash the zucchini and use a spiralizer to make the zucchini noodles. Peel the garlic and chop it.

2. Combine the cilantro, chopped garlic clove, nutmeg, and white pepper together in a mixing bowl.

3. Sprinkle the zucchini noodles with the spice mixture.

4. Pour the chicken stock in the pressure cooker and sauté the liquid on the manual mode until it is become to boil.

5. Add the zucchini noodles and wine vinegar and stir the mixture gently.

6. Cook for 3 minutes on the "Sauté" mode. Remove the zucchini noodles from the pressure cooker and serve.

Nutrition: calories 28, fat 0.7, fiber 1, carbs 3.94, protein 2

Romano Zucchini

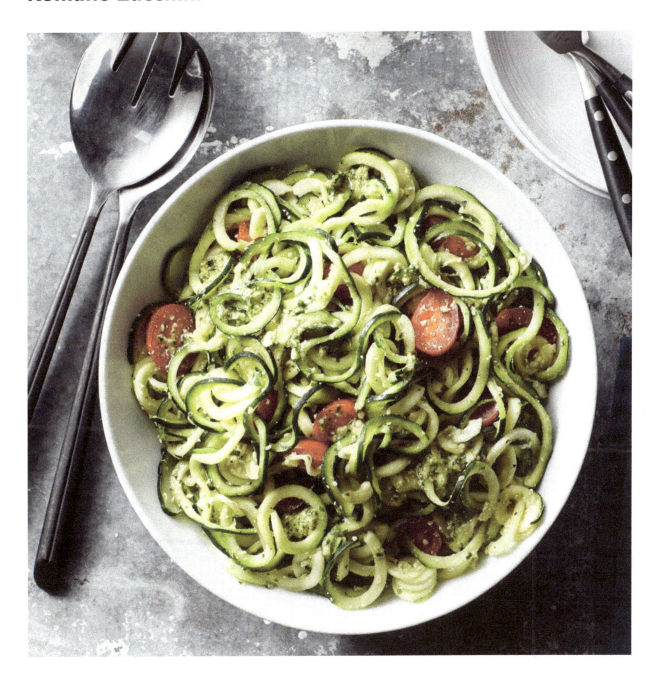

Prep time: 10 minutes

Cooking time: 30 minutes

Servings: 6

Ingredients:

- 1 pound yellow zucchini
- 3 tablespoons minced garlic
- ½ cup coconut flour
- 3 tablespoons olive oil
- 3 eggs
- ¼ cup of coconut milk
- 7 ounces Romano cheese
- 1 teaspoon salt

Directions:

1. Wash the zucchini and slice them. Combine the minced garlic and salt together and stir the mixture.

2. Combine the minced garlic mixture and zucchini slices together and mix well. Add the eggs in the mixing bowl and whisk the mixture.

3. Add coconut milk and coconut flour. Stir it carefully until combined. Grate the Romano cheese and add it to the egg mixture and mix.

4. Pour the olive oil in the pressure cooker and preheat it. Dip the sliced zucchini in the egg mixture.

5. Transfer the dipped zucchini in the pressure cooker and cook the dish on the "Sauté" mode for 2 minutes on each side.

6. When the dish is cooked, remove it from the pressure cooker, drain any excess fat using a paper towel, and serve.

Nutrition: calories 301, fat 21.6, fiber 5.1, carbs 12.5, protein 16

Salty Spaghetti Squash

Prep time: 10 minutes

Cooking time: 6 minutes

Servings: 3

Ingredients:

- 2 cups spaghetti squash, cubed
- 2 tablespoons butter
- ½ teaspoon salt
- 1 cup water, for cooking

Directions:

1. Pour water and insert the steamer rack in the instant pot.

2. Arrange the spaghetti squash cubes in the instant pot and cook them on manual mode (high pressure) for 6 minutes.

3. Then make a quick pressure release and open the lid.

4. Transfer the cooked squash cube sin the serving plates and top them with butter and salt. Wait till butter and salt dissolve.

Nutrition value/serving: calories 89, fat 2, fiber 8.1, carbs 4.7, protein 0.5

Mozzarella Zucchini Casserole

Prep time: 10 minutes

Cooking time: 5 minutes

Servings: 4

Ingredients:

- 2 zucchini, sliced
- 1 tomato, sliced
- ½ cup kohlrabi, chopped
- ½ cup chicken broth
- 1 teaspoon salt
- 1 teaspoon ground paprika
- 1 tablespoon nuts, chopped
- ½ cup Mozzarella, chopped
- ½ teaspoon sesame oil

Directions:

1. Brush the instant pot bowl with sesame oil.

2. Place the zucchini slices in the instant pot.

3. Then top them with sliced tomato and chopped kohlrabi.

4. After this, mix up together chicken broth, salt, and ground paprika.

5. Pour the liquid over the ingredients.

6. Then sprinkle the casserole mixture with nuts and Mozzarella.

7. Close the lid and cook the casserole on High pressure (manual mode) for 5 minutes.

8. When the time is over, make a quick pressure release.

9. Cool the cooked casserole to the room temperature.

Nutrition value/serving: calories 57, fat 2.8, fiber 2.3, carbs 6, protein 3.7

Button Beans Casserole

Prep time: 10 minutes

Cooking time: 20 minutes

Servings: 6

Ingredients:

- 1-pound green beans, chopped
- 1 cup button mushrooms, chopped
- 1 garlic clove, diced
- ½ white onion, diced
- 1 teaspoon butter
- 1/3 cup heavy cream
- ½ teaspoon salt
- 2 tablespoons almond meal
- 1 teaspoon Italian seasonings
- 1 teaspoon coconut oil, melted

Directions:

1. Toss butter in the instant pot and melt it on sauté mode.

2. Add onion and cook it for 2 minutes.

3. Then stir it and add mushrooms.

4. Cook the mixture for 2 minutes more.

5. Stir the ingredients again and add garlic clove, green beans, and salt. Mix up well.

6. In the mixing bowl combine together coconut oil, Italian seasonings, almond meal, and cream.

7. Pour the liquid over the casserole mixture and close the lid.

8. Cook it on sauté mode for 16 minutes.

Nutrition value/serving: calories 79, fat 5.2, fiber 3.2, carbs 7.5, protein 2.5

Ground Zucchini Casserole

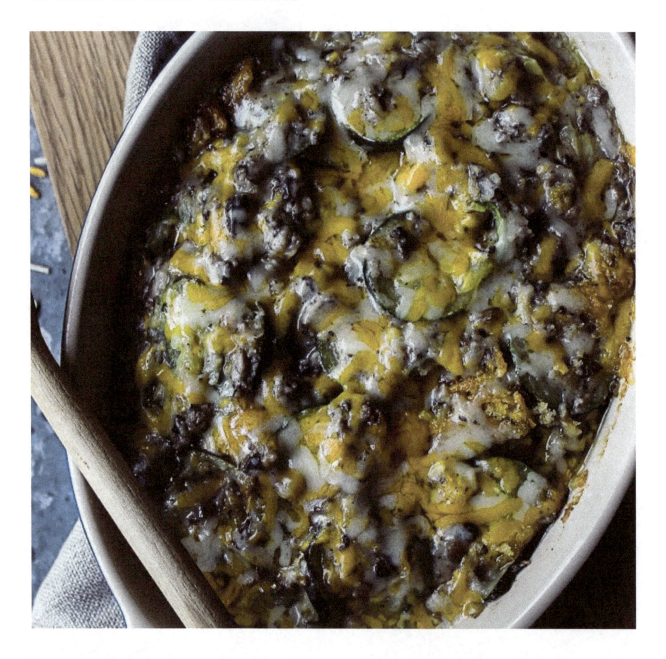

Prep time: 10 minutes

Cooking time: 5 minutes

Servings: 3

Ingredients:

- 7 oz spaghetti squash, chopped
- 1 zucchini, grated
- ½ cup Cheddar cheese
- 1 tablespoon cream cheese
- ½ teaspoon salt
- 1 teaspoon ground black pepper
- 1 cup water, for cooking

Directions:

1. Make the layer of spaghetti squash in the baking pan and top it with grated zucchini.

2. After this, sprinkle the zucchini with Cheddar cheese.

3. In the mixing bowl combine together cream cheese, salt, and ground black pepper.

4. Spread the mixture over the Cheddar cheese.

5. Pour water and insert the trivet in the instant pot.

6. Place the baking pan with casserole in the instant pot and cook it on manual mode (high pressure) for 6 minutes.

7. Then make a quick pressure release.

8. Let the cooked casserole rest for 10 minutes before serving.

Nutrition value/serving: calories 120, fat 7.9, fiber 0.9, carbs 7.5, protein 6.2

Almons and Mozzarella Zucchini Strips

Prep time: 10 minutes

Cooking time: 8 minutes

Servings: 2

Ingredients:

- 1 zucchini, trimmed
- 1/3 cup Mozzarella, shredded
- 1 teaspoon avocado oil

- 1 tablespoon almond meal

- ¼ teaspoon salt

Directions:

1. Cut the zucchini into the strips and sprinkle them with salt and almond meal.

2. Then heat up the instant pot on sauté mode for 2-3 minutes.

3. Add avocado oil.

4. Arrange the zucchini strips in one layer in the instant pot and cook them for 2 minutes from each side or until they are light brown.

5. Repeat the same steps with remaining zucchini strips (if you use small instant and can't arrange all vegetables per one time of cooking).

6. Then top the cooked zucchini strips with Mozzarella and close the lid.

7. Cook the side dish on sauté mode for 3 minutes or until the cheese is melted.

Nutrition value/serving: calories 49, fat 2.8, fiber 1.6, carbs 4.2, protein 3.2

Cabbage Rice

Prep time: 10 minutes

Cooking time: 35 minutes

Servings: 5

Ingredients:

- 1 ½ cup white cabbage, shredded
- 1 teaspoon salt
- 1 cup of coconut milk
- 1 teaspoon ground turmeric
- 1 white onion, diced
- 1 tablespoon coconut oil

Directions:

1. In the mixing bowl combine together salt and shredded cabbage. Leave the vegetables for 5 minutes.

2. Meanwhile, heat up the instant pot bowl on sauté mode for 2 minutes.

3. Add coconut oil and diced onion.

4. Cook the onion for 3 minutes.

5. Then stir it with the help of the spatula and add cabbage.

6. After this, in the bowl combine together ground turmeric and coconut milk.

7. When the liquid starts to be yellow, pour it over the cabbage.

8. Stir the cabbage and close the lid.

9. Cook the cabbage rice on sauté mode for 30 minutes. Stir ti from time to time to avoid burning.

Nutrition value/serving: calories 149, fat 14.2, fiber 2.2, carbs 6.2, protein 1.6

Cheddar Creamy Gratin

Prep time: 5 minutes

Cooking time: 7 minutes

Servings: 2

Ingredients:

- 1 cup turnip, sliced
- 1/3 cup heavy cream
- ¼ teaspoon salt
- ¼ teaspoon dried sage
- 1 teaspoon butter
- 1/3 teaspoon garlic powder
- ½ cup Cheddar cheese, shredded

Directions:

1. Toss butter in the instant pot and melt it on sauté mode (approx.2-3 minutes).

2. Then add sliced turnip and cook it on sauté mode for 1 minute from each side.

3. Sprinkle the vegetables with salt, dried sage, and garlic powder.

4. Then add heavy cream.

5. Top the turnip with Cheddar cheese and close the lid.

6. Cook the meal on manual mode (high pressure) for 3 minutes. Then make a quick pressure release.

Nutrition value/serving: calories 220, fat 18.8, fiber 1.3, carbs 5.5, protein 8.1

White Onion Rings

Prep time: 10 minutes

Cooking time: 5 minutes

Servings: 4

Ingredients:

- 1 big white onion
- 1 egg, beaten
- 1 teaspoon cream cheese
- 2 oz Parmesan, grated
- 2 tablespoons almond meal
- 1 tablespoon butter

Directions:

1. Trim and peel the onion.

2. Then slice it roughly and separate every onion slice into the rings.

3. In the mixing bowl combine together Parmesan and almond meal.

4. Then take a separated bowl and mix up cream cheese and egg in it.

5. Dip the onion rings in the egg mixture and then coat well in cheese mixture.

6. Toss butter in the instant pot and melt it on sauté mode.

7. Then arrange the onion rings in the melted butter in one layer.

8. Cook the onion rings for 2 minutes from each side on sauté mode.

Nutrition value/serving: calories 122, fat 8.8, fiber 1.2, carbs 4.8, protein 7.1

Rosemary Halves

Prep time: 10 minutes

Cooking time: 10 minutes

Servings: 4

Ingredients:

- 3 cups radish, trimmed
- 1 tablespoon olive oil
- 1 teaspoon dried rosemary
- ½ teaspoon salt

Directions:

1. Cut the radishes into the halves and sprinkle with salt.

2. In the shallow bowl whisk together olive oil and dried rosemary.

3. After this, sprinkle the radish halves with fragrant oil and shake the vegetables well.

4. Transfer the radishes in the instant pot and cook the on sauté mode for 10 minutes.

5. Stir the vegetables every 2 minutes.

Nutrition value/serving: calories 45, fat 3.6, fiber 1.5, carbs 3.2, protein 0.6

Sweet Baby Carrot

Prep time: 10 minutes

Cooking time: 4 minutes

Servings: 4

Ingredients:

- 1 cup baby carrot
- 1 tablespoon Erythritol
- ½ teaspoon dried thyme
- 2 tablespoons butter, melted
- 1 cup water, for cooking

Directions:

1. Wash the baby carrot carefully and trim if needed.
2. Then pour water in the instant pot and insert the trivet,

3. Put the prepared baby carrots in the baking pan.

4. Add dried thyme, Erythritol, and butter. Mix up the vegetables well and place over the trivet.

5. Close the lid.

6. Cook the carrot for 4 minutes on manual mode (high pressure).

7. When the time is over make a quick pressure release.

Nutrition value/serving: calories 69, fat 5.8, fiber 1.1, carbs 7.8, protein 0.6

Chili Zucchini Bowl

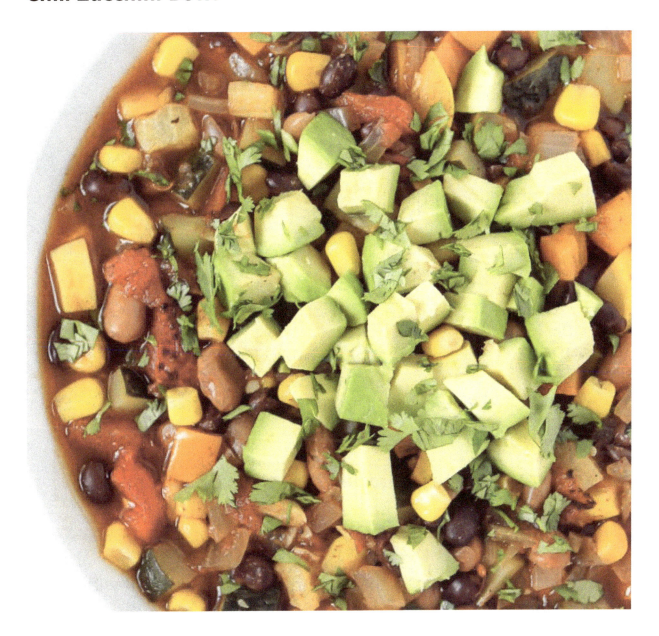

Prep time: 5 minutes

Cooking time: 3 minutes

Servings: 4

Ingredients:

- 2 zucchini, chopped
- 1 teaspoon olive oil
- ½ teaspoon chili flakes
- ½ teaspoon paprika
- 2 oz Feta, crumbled

Directions:

1. Place olive oil, zucchini, chili flakes, and paprika in the instant pot.

2. Stir the ingredients gently and close the lid.

3. Cook zucchini on sauté mode for 2 minutes.

4. Then open the lid and mix up them well with the help of the spatula.

5. Keep cooking zucchini for 1 minute more.

6. Transfer the cooked zucchini into the serving bowls and top with feta cheese.

Nutrition value/serving: calories 64, fat 4.4, fiber 1.2, carbs 4, protein 3.2

Thyme Asparagus

Prep time: 5 minutes

Cooking time: 5 minute

Servings: 2

Ingredients:

- 6 oz asparagus, trimmed
- ¼ teaspoon dried thyme
- ¼ teaspoon salt
- ¼ teaspoon ground black pepper
- ¼ teaspoon dried oregano
- ¼ teaspoon ground nutmeg
- 2 tablespoons butter
- ¼ cup chicken broth

Directions:

1. In the mixing bowl combine together dried thyme, salt, ground black pepper, oregano, and nutmeg.

2. Then put the asparagus in the instant pot.

3. Sprinkle the vegetables with spice mixture. Stir them gently.

4. Then add butter and chicken broth.

5. Close the lid and cook asparagus on manual mode (high pressure) for 5 minutes.

6. Then make the quick pressure release, open the lid, and shake the asparagus gently.

Nutrition value/serving: calories 127, fat 11.9, fiber 2.1, carbs 3.9, protein 2.7

Minced Radish

Prep time: 8 minutes

Cooking time: 3 minutes

Servings: 3

Ingredients:

- 1 ½ cup radish, sliced
- ½ teaspoon minced garlic
- 1 teaspoon sesame oil
- ¼ cup Monterey Jack cheese, shredded
- ¼ cup heavy cream
- 1 tablespoon cream cheese

Directions:

1. Put radish minced garlic, sesame oil, heavy cream, and cream cheese in the instant pot.

2. Mix up the radish mixture well.

3. Then top it with shredded cheese and close the lid.

4. Cook the radish for 3 minutes on Manual mode (high pressure).

5. Then make a quick pressure release.

Nutrition value/serving: calories 105, fat 9.3, fiber 0.9, carbs 2.6, protein 3.2

Peppery Cubes

Prep time: 10 minutes

Cooking time: 3 minutes

Servings: 6

Ingredients:

- 1-pound turnip, cubed
- 1 teaspoon salt
- ½ teaspoon ground black pepper
- 1 teaspoon avocado oil
- 1 cup water, for cooking

Directions:

1. Pour water and insert the steamer rack in the instant pot.

2. In the mixing bowl mix up together turnip cubes, salt, and ground black pepper.

3. Sprinkle the vegetables with avocado oil and place them in the steamer rack.

4. Close and seal the lid.

5. Cook the turnip on Manual mode (high pressure) for 3 minutes.

6. Then allow the natural pressure release for 5 minutes.

Nutrition value/serving: calories 23, fat 0.2, fiber 1.4, carbs 5, protein 0.7

Pecan Salad

Prep time: 10 minutes

Cooking time: 2 minutes

Servings: 2

Ingredients:

- 2 cups kale, chopped
- ½ cup fresh cilantro, chopped
- 1 pecan, chopped
- ½ teaspoon ground paprika
- ¼ teaspoon salt
- 1 tablespoon avocado oil
- 1 cucumber, chopped
- 1 cup water, for cooking

Directions:

1. Pour water and insert the steamer rack in the instant pot.

2. Place the kale in the steamer. Close and seal the lid.

3. Cook the greens for 2 minutes on Manual mode (high pressure).

4. Then make a quick pressure release and transfer the kale in the salad bowl.

5. Add chopped cilantro, pecan, and cucumber.

6. After this, sprinkle the salad with ground paprika, salt, and avocado oil.

7. Mix up the salad well.

Nutrition value/serving: calories 98, fat 6.2, fiber 3.1, carbs 9.2, protein 3

Cheese Gnocchi

Prep time: 15 minutes

Cooking time: 8 minutes

Servings: 6

Ingredients:

- 2 cups cauliflower, boiled
- 1 egg yolk
- ¼ cup coconut flour
- ½ cup almond meal
- 1 tablespoon cream cheese
- 2 oz Parmesan, grated
- 1 teaspoon dried basil
- 2 tablespoons butter

Directions:

1. Place the boiled cauliflower in the food processor and blend it until smooth.

2. Then add egg yolk, coconut flour, almond meal, cream cheese, and grated Parmesan.

3. Blend the cauliflower mixture for 15 seconds more.

4. Then transfer the mixture on the chopping board and knead it into the ball.

5. Then cut the dough ball into 3 parts.

6. After this, make 3 logs from the dough.

7. Cut the logs into the small gnocchi with the help of the cutter.

8. Toss the butter in the instant pot and melt it for 2 minutes on sauté mode.

9. Add dried basil and bring the butter to boil (it will take around 1 minute).

10. After this, add prepared gnocchi and cook them for 5 minutes. Stir the gnocchi from time to time.

Nutrition value/serving: calories 155, fat 11.7, fiber 3.8, carbs 7.3, protein 7.1

Purple Cabbage Steaks

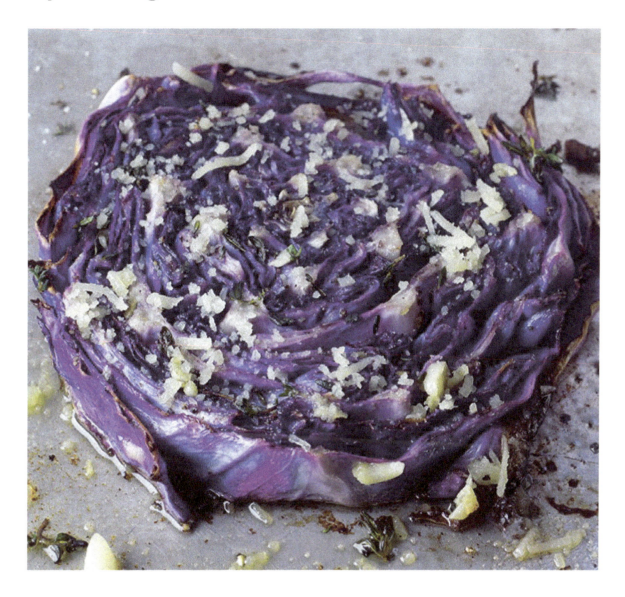

Prep time: 10 minutes

Cooking time: 4 minutes

Servings: 4

Ingredients:

- 10 oz purple cabbage
- 1 teaspoon apple cider vinegar
- 1 teaspoon olive oil
- ½ teaspoon salt
- ½ teaspoon lemon juice
- 1 cup water, for cooking

Directions:

1. Cut the purple cabbage into 4 cabbage steaks.

2. Pour water and insert the steamer rack in the instant pot.

3. Place the cabbage steaks on the rack and close the lid.

4. Cook the vegetables for 4 minutes on Manual mode (high pressure).

5. Then allow the natural pressure release for 5 minutes.

6. Place the cabbage steaks in the serving plates.

7. In the shallow bowl whisk together apple cider vinegar, olive oil, salt, and lemon juice.

8. Sprinkle every cabbage steak with apple cider vinegar mixture.

Nutrition value/serving: calories 28, fat 1.3, fiber 1.8, carbs 4.1, protein 0.9

Cauliflower and Goat Cheese

Prep time: 15 minutes

Cooking time: 5 minutes

Servings: 3

Ingredients:

- 1 ½ cup cauliflower, chopped
- ½ teaspoon salt
- 2 oz Goat cheese, crumbled
- 1 tablespoon cream cheese
- 1 cup water, for cooking

Directions:

1. Pour water and insert the steamer rack in the instant pot.

2. Place the cauliflower in the steamer rack and close the lid.

3. Cook the vegetables on manul mode (high pressure) for 5 minutes. Make a quick pressure release.

4. Place the cooked cauliflower in the food processor and blend it until smooth.

5. Transfer the cauliflower into the bowl. Add salt and cream cheese. Mix up the cauliflower mass well.

6. Place the cooked meal on the plate and top with goat cheese.

Nutrition value/serving: calories 110, fat 7.9, fiber 1.3, carbs 3.2, protein 7

Mushrooms and Fall Vegetables

Prep time: 10 minutes

Cooking time: 8 minutes

Servings: 5

Ingredients:

- 1 cup mushrooms, chopped
- 1 cup zucchini, chopped
- 1/2 cup bell pepper, chopped
- 1 eggplant, chopped
- 3 tablespoons butter
- ½ teaspoon salt
- 1 teaspoon dried basil
- 1 teaspoon dried thyme
- ½ teaspoon ground black pepper
- ½ teaspoon cayenne pepper

- 1 cup water, for cooking

Directions:

1. Pour water and insert the trivet in the instant pot.

2. Put all vegetables in the instant pot baking pan.

3. Sprinkle them with salt, dried basil, thyme, ground black pepper, and cayenne pepper.

4. Mix up the vegetables and top with butter.

5. Arrange the baking pan with vegetables in the instant pot.

6. Close the lid and cook the side dish for 8 minutes on Manual mode (high pressure).

7. Make a quick pressure release.

Nutrition value/serving: calories 96, fat 7.2, fiber 4, carbs 7.9, protein 1.9

Garlic Broccoli

Prep time: 10 minutes

Cooking time: 1 minute

Servings: 2

Ingredients:

- 1 cup broccoli florets
- ½ teaspoon garlic, diced
- ¼ teaspoon salt
- 1 teaspoon sesame oil
- 1 cup water, for cooking

Directions:

1. Pour water and insert the steamer rack in the instant pot.

2. Place the broccoli florets in the steamer rack and close the lid.

3. Cook the vegetables on Manual mode (high pressure) for 1 minute.

4. Then make a quick pressure release and transfer the cooked broccoli florets in the serving plates.

5. Sprinkle vegetables with garlic, salt, and sesame oil.

Nutrition value/serving: calories 37, fat 2.4, fiber 1.2, carbs 3.3, protein 1.3

Tots with Broccoli

Prep time: 10 minutes

Cooking time: 5 minutes

Servings: 4

Ingredients:

- 1 cup broccoli, shredded
- ¼ cup Cheddar cheese, shredded
- ¼ teaspoon garlic powder
- ¼ teaspoon salt
- 2 tablespoon almond meal
- ¼ teaspoon ground black pepper
- 1 teaspoon coconut oil
- 1 teaspoon dried dill

Directions:

1. In the mixing bowl combine together shredded broccoli, cheese, garlic powder, salt, almond meal, ground black pepper, and dried dill.

2. Mix up the mixture with the help of the spoon until homogenous.

3. After this, make the small tots from the mixture.

4. Heat up instant pot bowl on sauté mode for 3 minutes.

5. Then toss coconut oil and melt it (appx.1 minute).

6. Then arrange the tots in the instant pot in one layer and cook tots for 1 minute from each side.

Nutrition value/serving: calories 65, fat 5.1, fiber 1, carbs 2.6, protein 3.1

Vegetable Fritters

Prep time: 10 minutes

Cooking time: 6 minutes

Servings: 4

Ingredients:

- ½ cup turnip, boiled
- ½ cup cauliflower, boiled
- 1 egg, beaten
- 1 teaspoon dried parsley
- 3 tablespoons coconut flour
- 1 teaspoon avocado oil
- 1/3 teaspoon salt
- 1 teaspoon ground turmeric

Directions:

1. Mash turnip and cauliflower with the help of the potato masher.

2. Then add egg, dried parsley, coconut flour, salt, and ground turmeric in the mashed mixture and stir well.

3. Make the medium side fritters and place them in the instant pot.

4. Add avocado oil.

5. Cook the fritters on sauté mode for 3 minutes from each side.

Nutrition value/serving: calories 50, fat 1.9, fiber 3, carbs 6, protein 2.6

Pressured Asparagus

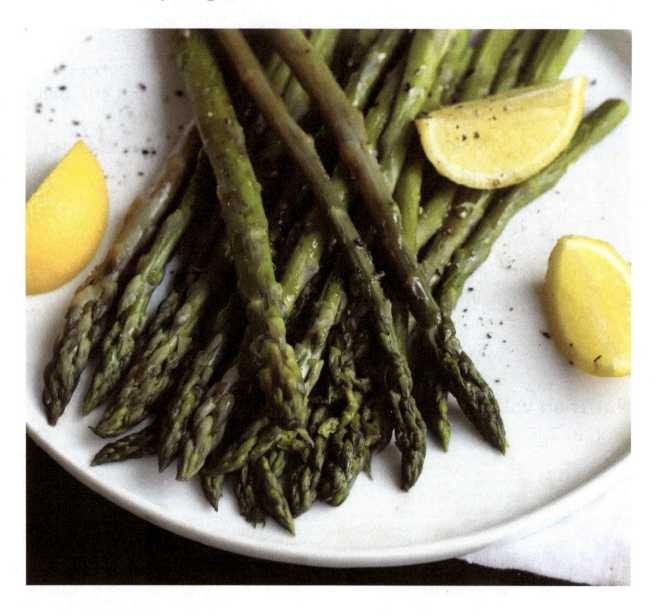

Prep time: 5 minutes

Cooking time: 1 minute

Servings: 2

Ingredients:

- 6 oz asparagus, chopped
- ¼ teaspoon salt
- 1 cup water, for cooking

Directions:

1. Pour water and insert the steamer rack in the instant pot.
2. Place the chopped asparagus in the steamer rack and close the lid.
3. Cook the vegetables on Manual (high pressure) for 1 minute.
4. Then make a quick pressure release and open the lid.
5. Sprinkle the asparagus with salt.

Nutrition value/serving: calories 17, fat 0.1, fiber 1.8, carbs 3.3, protein 1.9

Roasted Cider Steak

Prep time: 10 minutes

Cooking time: 4 minutes

Servings: 2

Ingredients:

- 8 oz cauliflower
- 1 teaspoon olive oil
- ½ teaspoon apple cider vinegar
- ¼ teaspoon chili flakes
- ¼ teaspoon salt
- ¼ teaspoon onion powder
- ¼ teaspoon ground turmeric
- 1 cup water, for cooking

Directions:

1. Cut the cauliflower into medium steaks.

2. In the shallow bowl combine together olive oil, apple cider vinegar, chili flakes, salt, onion powder, and ground turmeric.

3. Then brush the cauliflower steaks with oily mixture form both sides.

4. Pour water and insert the trivet in the instant pot.

5. Arrange the cauliflower steaks in the instant pot in one layer.

6. Cook the vegetables for 4 minutes on manual mode (high pressure).

7. Then make a quick pressure release.

8. Cool the cauliflower steaks for 2-5 minutes before serving.

Nutrition value/serving: calories 51, fat 2.5, fiber 2.9, carbs 6.5, protein 2.3

Cayenne Pepper Green Beans

Prep time: 10 minutes

Cooking time: 3 minutes

Servings: 4

Ingredients:

- 2 cups green beans, chopped
- 1 teaspoon cayenne pepper
- 1 tablespoon nut oil
- ¼ teaspoon salt
- 1 cup water, for coking

Directions:

1. Pour water and insert the steamer rack in the instant pot.

2. Place the green beans in the steamer rack.

3. Cook the vegetables for 3 minutes on Manual mode (high pressure).

4. Make a quick pressure release and cool the green beans in ice water for 4 minutes.

5. Transfer the green beans in the mixing bowl and sprinkle with nut oil and salt. Mix up the beans well.

Nutrition value/serving: calories 48, fat 3.5, fiber 2, carbs 4.2, protein 1.1

Conclusion

Being an excellent solution both for immediate pot beginners and knowledgeable instant pot customers this instantaneous pot cookbook elevates your day-to-day cooking. It makes you resemble a professional and also cook like a pro. Thanks to the Instant Pot part, this cookbook aids you with preparing easy and also tasty dishes for any type of budget plan. Satisfy every person with passionate dinners, nutritious morning meals, sweetest desserts, and fun snacks.
No matter if you cook for one or prepare larger portions-- there's a service for any feasible food preparation circumstance. Improve your methods on exactly how to cook in the most reliable way utilizing just your instant pot, this cookbook, and also some patience to find out quickly.
Practical tips as well as tricks are subtly integrated into every dish to make your family demand brand-new dishes time and time again. Vegetarian alternatives, options for meat-eaters as well as extremely pleasing suggestions to unite the entire family members at the very same table. Eating in your home is a shared experience, and also it can be so good to meet entirely at the end of the day. Master your Instant Pot and take advantage of this brand-new experience beginning today!